The Ultimate Guide To Smoothie Diet

How To Detox Your Body, Lose Weight And Rejuvenate With Top 15 Best Smoothie Recipes

Elizabeth Grace

Table of Contents

Introduction

I want to thank you and congratulate you for purchasing the book, *"The Ultimate Guide to Smoothie Diet: How to Detox Your Body. Lose Weight and Rejuvenate with Top 15 Best Smoothie Recipes"*.

This book contains proven steps and strategies on how to start a smoothie diet.

Making smoothies are convenient and smart way to ensure that you are consuming enough fruits and vegetables during the day. Most people find it difficult to eat several servings of fruits and vegetables in one sitting but it only take a couple of minutes to sip smoothies.

Smoothies offer pure nutrition. You tend to get higher amount of nutrients with each serving compared to fresh juice. Drinking smoothies are also better for your digestion. Smoothies are also cheap and easy to make. You can drink smoothies in place of a meal and not feel hungry for several hours.

You can tailor your smoothie to accommodate your diet. Try to mix and experiment on different ingredients for your smoothie or try the recipes in this book.

Thanks again for purchasing this book, I hope you enjoy it!

Chapter 1: What is Smoothie?

Smoothies are unlike regular juice or beverage. Fresh juice is made by extracting the liquid from fruits and vegetables and leaving the pulp behind. Smoothies are made by blending the whole fruit.

A glass of fresh fruit juice can only amount to one serving of fruits and vegetables no matter what kind of produce is used. Smoothies are much more nutritious and contain more fiber, vitamins and carbohydrates. One glass of smoothie can be filling and satisfying.

Benefits of smoothies

Eating the recommended amount of fruits and vegetables every day can be difficult for most people. Drinking smoothies is an easier way of consuming your vegetables.

Easy and convenient

Blending a smoothie usually takes less time than preparing your meals. This enables you to do other things instead. Smoothies are also more convenient and portable to carry.

Children like smoothies

Kids are notorious for being picky eaters but they tend to like smoothies most especially if you add sweet fruits for flavor.

For weight loss

There are a lot of weight loss programs that recommend replacing meals with drinks. You can provide your body with the needed vitamins and minerals by drinking smoothies without the added calories of sugar and artificial ingredients.

Improved digestion

Constipation and indigestion can be very uncomfortable. You can make it easier for your stomach to digest the food by blending it first.

It is delicious

Drinking healthy smoothies can also taste good. There are many great tasting fruits and vegetables to choose from and you can certainly find one that you like.

Detox

You can easily add detoxifying ingredients like kale and dandelion greens into your smoothies to make your own detox drink.

Improve your athletic performance

You can provide your body with the needed nutrients to excel in any competition by drinking smoothie. It is easier for the body to absorb the nutrients from a smoothie than a regular meal.

Beauty benefits

You can achieve radiant skin and silkier hair just by drinking smoothies. Supply your body with vitamins and nutrients needed to make your skin glow.

Strengthen your immune system

You can reduce the risk of common illnesses by improving your immune system. Most fruits and vegetables used for smoothies contain vitamin C which can boost your immune system.

Meal flexibility

Smoothies can be consumed at any time of the day. You can also substitute it for snack or meal when you don't have enough time to make your own meal.

Give you a sense of empowerment

You can feel empowered by taking control of the foods that you consume. Leading a healthy lifestyle can also make you experience a new sense of well being and happiness which can improve your mood.

You can get creative

People who regularly include smoothies in their diet find it enjoyable to mix various ingredients and experiment on different flavors.

Brain boost

Skip processed food and opt for healthy smoothies instead. Drinking smoothies made from fruits and vegetables can improve your focus and memory. It can also drastically reduce brain fog and tiredness.

Reduce cravings

One of the reasons why people crave certain food is because their body is not getting enough vitamins and nutrients. Unfortunately, most people supply these cravings with unhealthy alternatives. Replace these foods with naturally sweet and delicious smoothie instead.

Explore healthy ingredients

There is a vast array of healthy ingredients that you can use in a smoothie. You can choose your basic fruit and vegetables then add herbs, spices and natural sweeteners.

Basic types of Smoothies

The fruit smoothie

This is typically made from any type of fruits with healthy sweeteners like honey, butter or even spices.

Green smoothies

Green smoothies include green leafy vegetables. You can easily turn any fruit smoothie into a green smoothie by adding kale or spinach.

Thick fruit smoothie

A fruit smoothie can easily turn into a complete meal by increasing it healthy carbohydrate content. This will naturally thicken the smoothie which can fill you for a longer time. You can make a thick fruit smoothie by adding good carbohydrates like oats, tofu and buckwheat.

Green thick smoothie

Green thick smoothies are usually made with 2 cups of greens and 1 cup of carbohydrates. Green thick smoothies contain the right amount of carbohydrates to satisfy you.

Chapter 2: Smoothie Tricks and Tips

Smoothies are relatively easy to prepare. Keep these tips in mind when blending your own smoothie.

- Add the ice last. This way, you can make your smoothies frosty and icy. Adding the ice at the beginning of the blending process can only make it watery.

- Use fresh ingredients as much as possible. Fresh fruits and vegetables have natural flavors and contain a higher amount of vitamins and nutrients.

- Freeze the banana. If you like adding bananas into your smoothies, remember that it is best to use frozen bananas. Store your overripe bananas in the freezer and use it for smoothies. Make sure that you peel and chop the bananas before blending.

- Add your fresh fruits towards the end of the blending process. Adding fresh fruits to a frozen fruit combination really brings out the flavor. You should also blend the fresh fruit minimally as much as possible.

- No to soy and citrus. If you want to make a soy-based smoothie, it is best to choose non citrus fruit juices with it. Orange and soymilk do not taste well together and can even curdle. Opt for blackberries, blueberries and bananas instead for soy based smoothies. Adding coconut water to soymilk also adds a hint of tropical flavor.

- Add acid for tartness. Fruits like blueberries are healthy and delicious but do not contain much acid. Pair it with acid fruits like orange juice to compliment it.

- Use natural sugar. You can skip adding refined sugar in your smoothies since the fruit juice and natural fruits provide enough sweetness. Fruit juices that contain high fructose include pear juice, apple juice, grape juice and pomegranate juice.

- Don't be afraid to get creative. Add less common smoothie ingredients like kiwi, papaya, coconut meat, lychees, watermelon and aloe vera into your drinks.

- Use less liquid first then adjust later on. It is better to use less liquid at the beginning and add more later on if it becomes necessary.

- Do not use crusty fruit. If you cannot eat the fruit on its own, it cannot taste good in a smoothie. Throw away any old and white crusted fruit since it is usually flavorless.

- Add a probiotic boost to your smoothies. Adding soy and yogurt to your drinks gives it a nutritional boost. You can use plain yogurt to add a tangy flavor. Lemon yogurt also tastes delicious in smoothies.

- Try organic produce. Organic fruits have more flavor than conventional fruit.

- Use fresh frozen fruit to have the best consistency. The best consistency for a fruit smoothie is usually achieved by using two thirds of frozen ingredients. Freezing fruits are easy and simple. You just need to cut it to smaller pieces before blending.

- The best ingredients to add for a better texture include nut butter, avocado, oatmeal, coconut oil and Greek yogurt. You can easily turn an ordinary smoothie to a creamy delight by adding a tablespoon of nut butter. Avocados are best used for green smoothies. You can add the avocado during the last minute of blending. Cooked oatmeal can work with sweet and savory smoothies. Greek yogurt provides a great texture to your drink and coconut oil adds tropical creaminess to the mixture.

- Use local and in-season fruits. Using different fruits and vegetables can keep your smoothies interesting. It also enables you to get the different nutrients. Also, take advantage of in-season fruits since they are cheaper and taste better.

- Use spices. Different spices can enhance the flavor of the drink. The most popular spices include cinnamon, ginger, cayenne pepper and nutmeg.

- Add protein. A green smoothie can turn into a protein shake by adding few scoops of whey protein. Protein shakes are popular for people who want to gain muscle.

- Adding healthy fat like hemp oil, coconut and flax can keep you satiated for a longer time.

- Add a little bit of salt. Adding high quality salt can improve the taste of your smoothies and also add minerals. Choose Celtic salt, Himalayan salt or Redmond salt for best results.

- Use the seeds. Using seeds like flax, chia and help can boost the nutrient content of you smoothies. You can soak the seeds in water to make a gel.

- Try fruit flavored ice cubes. You can use coconut water ice cubes and banana ice cubes. Just chop the fruits into smaller pieces and place it a bag before freezing it.

Chapter 3: Smoothies FAQ

The process of making smoothies has been practiced for a long time.

Here are some of the frequently asked questions about smoothies:

How to prepare the ingredients?

Make sure to peel the tips and remove the seeds and core of the fruits and vegetables before blending them. The exceptions are raspberries and strawberries where the seeds are difficult to remove. Any fruit that has small seeds can also be blended whole.

How thick should the smoothie be?

Smoothies should be pulpy and thicker than regular juice. Smoothies with wheat and starch tend to be very thick. You can dilute the smoothie with water, juice or milk. You can also add fruits and vegetables that have high water content like cucumber and watermelon. How thick the smoothie should be is a personal preference. Some people like very thick consistency while others like it thinner which makes it easier to drink from a straw.

Do I need to add sweetener?

Most smoothies are already sweet enough because of the fruits but you can also add honey or maple syrup. If the smoothie tastes too sweet, you can add lime or lemon juice to balance the flavor. Adjust the taste of the smoothie before you drink it since its natural flavor tends to become more pronounced the longer it is left to stand.

How long can I keep the smoothie?

Smoothies are best drunk as soon as they are made because the vitamin count usually decreases when it is left standing. Once the smoothie is exposed to air, the fruit can oxidize and can turn to brown. Citrus flavors also become more pronounced and can overpower the other flavors.

Why does yogurt and blueberry smoothie curdle?

Smoothies that are made with citrus, pineapple and blueberries should be consumed as soon as possible if it is combined with dairy products. The longer it stands, the thicker it gets and produces a curdled appearance. This is a chemical reaction of the protein in dairy products and the casein content of the fruit. You can also prepare the smoothie in advance and add the milk just before serving.

How to remove froth from the smoothie?

Fruits like apples and pears produce a thicker froth than other ingredients. It is best to remove the froth by skimming it off using a spoon. You can also use a straw to drink the smoothie from the bottom of the glass.

Can I use any combination of fruits and vegetables?

Yes. Just remember to search for fresh ingredients as much as possible to have a delicious and great tasting smoothie. It is also best to avoid combining strong flavors since they can overpower each other. Fruits that have dense flesh like avocado and mango are best paired with fruits that are juicier like cucumber and oranges.

Is adding leafy green vegetables make the smoothie taste weird?

As long as you use 40% vegetables and 60% fruits, you will not even notice the taste of the vegetables. The fruits usually mask the taste. Bananas are usually used as a sweetener for green smoothies.

How do I clean the blender?

The easiest way to clean your blender is by rinsing it with warm water after each use. You

can also add water and let it soak until you are
ready to wash it.

Chapter 4: Lose Weight, Detox and Rejuvenate with Smoothies

Switching to a healthy lifestyle requires commitment and patience if you want to see results. Here are some of the tips on how you can incorporate smoothies in your lifestyle.

Setting realistic weight loss goals

Every good weight loss program has two parts which include food and physical activity. Drinking smoothies on a regular basis can help you consume fewer calories without feeling deprived and hungry. Smoothies also contain vitamins and nutrients which can give your body enough energy to perform more physical activity.

Setting your goals can make a difference between success and failure. Realistic plans can help motivate you. It also gives you a concrete plan as you transition to a healthier lifestyle. While it is okay to dream big, be sure to be smart in creating goals.

Writing you goals in paper can help you see the bigger picture. Set a specific time and place where you can do it and what you need to get started.

Have a measurable goal

Make sure that you can measure your goals. For example, how many days are you going to exercise and for how long? Track your progress by writing it down. You should also observe your diet. You can aim to drink one or two servings of smoothies a day.

Focus on what is relevant and attainable for you

Set goals that are within your capabilities and you also have to consider your limitations. Taking your fitness level and health condition into consideration can help you tailor a personal fitness program. A reasonable goal for most people is to lose 5-10% of their current weight. Losing one or two pounds a week is also achievable.

Consider the timing

Just like anything, timing is also crucial in making a difference between success and failure. Unfortunately, very few people can concentrate on just losing weight. Work, school and family duties can keep you busy all day long. Try to squeeze in few minutes of exercise a day. Making smoothies can also save time and help ensure that you are getting enough vegetables.

It is a good idea to make short-term and long-term goal. The short-term goals can help you motivated every day while the long-term goal can help you look at the bigger picture. Be sure that your short-term goals can help you achieve your long-term goals.

Be ready for setbacks

It is natural to experience setbacks. You can think of a plan to overcome these challenge in advance and help you stay on your course.

Reassess and adjust your goals as needed

You should be willing to change your goals if you want to progress. Remember that as your body can get use to a routine. Be ready to take larger challenges. Make sure to adjust your personal goals to fit your lifestyle.

Tips in avoiding cravings and temptations

People who are trying to eat healthy will experience cravings. Cravings can be defined as the unreasonable desire of a particular food.

Unfortunately, most cravings involve greasy, fried and sweet foods. These foods contain a large amount of processed ingredients which is bad for the body.

One of the best ways to avoid these cravings is to remove them from your pantry. Your body is always trying to attain balance. The cravings that you experience may be a sign that you need a particular vitamin or mineral. Here are some tips in reducing cravings.

Drink more water

Thirst can be easily mistaken for hunger. When your body lacks water, your body sends a message to the brain that you are near dehydration. This produces the feeling of thirst and can also manifest as mild hunger. Try to drink water first when you experience cravings and see if you are really just thirsty.

Sleep more

Most people are so busy that they don't have enough time for sleep. When you are tired, you tend to experience more stress. This can lead to blood sugar fluctuations and cravings.

Eat enough protein

You need to eat the right amount of protein to be healthy. Too much or too little protein can lead to cravings. Sugar cravings can also be associated with lack of protein. Try to add tofu to your smoothies to increase it protein content.

Get rid of the stimulants

Stimulants are very addictive. Your body tends to crave more and more sugar as you continue to consume it. Unfortunately, sugar is added at almost every packaged and it can be difficult to avoid them entirely. Stick to natural sweeteners like fruits and honey instead to satisfy your sweet tooth without spiking your blood sugar level.

Include dark leafy greens in your diet

Eating or drinking dark leafy green vegetables are the best way to nourish your body. Green vegetables are great to pair with any meal. You can also combine it with other ingredients to make a green smoothie.

Eat your food according to season

Eating foods that are in season can help balance your diet and give you the nutrients that you need. During spring, your body may crave for leafy greens and citrus fruits. In summer, you may like to indulge with cool fruits. In the fall, you can eat squash, onions and nuts and during winter, your body tends to crave for heat producing foods like oil and meat.

Do not use food as a substitute for anything

Most people use food as their outlet. Emotional eating is a real issue that needs to be addressed if you want to lose weight. Confront your emotional problems directly instead of using food to avoid it.

Drink your smoothie during your most intense craving

Drinking smoothies when your cravings hit can prevent you from giving in to temptation. Make a sweet smoothie instead and satisfy your taste buds without indulging in unhealthy food options.

Consume sufficient calories and healthy carbohydrates

Persistent cravings for sweet food are a common problem for most people. If you are eating whole foods and you are still craving sweets, it is possible that you are not getting enough amounts of calories or carbohydrates in your diet.

Severe calorie restriction can be detrimental to your health and can derail your efforts. You can still lose weight and satisfy your cravings by drinking smoothies that contain nutrients without too much calories.

Detox your body and feel rejuvenated

People who are feeling fatigued or struggling with skin problems and digestive problems should consider a detox program. Detox is a process that has been practiced for several centuries around the world. It is about giving the body enough nourishment and eliminating toxins. Detoxification can also help protect you from disease and strengthen your immune system. Here are some tips on how you can detoxify your body naturally.

Replace one meal with a smoothie

Your smoothie can contain a high amount of vitamins and minerals which can already count as a meal. Replacing one meal with a smoothie is not difficult and can help your body get rid of unhealthy substance.

Make sure that you use natural ingredients rather than buying premade concoction smoothie. This also jumps starts your weight loss process and can keep your digestive system working properly.

Eat organic foods when possible

As a general tip, fruits and vegetables that can be eaten with their skin should be bought organic. Choosing organic food can help you avoid harmful toxins. This is one of the simplest ways on how you can detoxify your body.

Be diligent in looking for healthier options and learn how to read the label correctly. Making healthy choices can help you get rid of toxins that you were previously consuming.

Get a good massage

You may think than massages are relaxing luxuries but it can also be a good detox for your body. If you want to remove toxins in your body, you have to opt for a massage that focuses on your main pressure points. Good detox massages include Swedish massage or a Sport massage.

You would want to have a massage that treats your deep muscles. When these pressure points are pressed, the toxins are released. Make sure that you only go to registered massage therapists. To make it more effective, drink a lot of water to flush the toxins out of your system.

Drink more water

Drinking more water is the cheapest way to detoxify your body. Make it a habit to keep a bottle of water at your desk to remind you to drink often. Water flushes toxins out of your body. It can also improve your digestive and circulatory system.

Replace coffee with green tea

A small amount of caffeine is okay but you should also be careful about the amount of coffee that you consume in a day. Green tea offers more antioxidants when it is taken it its natural form. It also provides you the natural boost that you need.

Sweat it out

Exercise is a part of a healthy lifestyle. Exercise is also a natural and effective way to cleanse the body of toxins. As you exercise, you can sweat the toxins out of your body. Exercise also improves digestion and circulation. Remember that a healthy exercise and clean diet is part of a good weight loss plan.

Eat more fiber

Fiber can boost your weight loss. The digestive track tends to hold to substances like toxins and preservatives from the food that you eat if it is not flushed out. This can make you feel bloated and tired.

Add several servings of fiber into your diet to ensure that your digestive system is working properly. Fruits and vegetables are great source of fiber. You can increase your fiber consumption by drinking smoothies.

Avoid environment that has toxins

Toxins in the environment can also affect you. These toxins include smog or bad air quality. Any type of chemical smoke is also bad for you. Avoid these environments as much as possible.

Switch to probiotics to remove bad bacteria

Probiotics are powerful substance that can naturally eliminate bad bacteria in your body. One of the most popular sources of probiotics is yogurt. It can keep you digestive tract functioning properly. Add yogurt into your smoothies to boost the probiotic content of you smoothies.

Chapter 5: 15 Smoothie Recipes

Here are some healthy and delicious smoothies recipes that can help you lose weight and feel energized.

1. Lean and Peachy Smoothie

This smoothie is made from peaches and blackberries which can provide you with a healthy dose of antioxidants.

½ cup low fat peach yogurt

½ cup peaches, frozen and roughly chopped

¼ cup unsweetened apple juice

1 cup frozen unsweetened blackberries

1 banana, frozen and thawed

Makes 1 serving

Pour the apple juice and yogurt in your blender. Add the blackberries, bananas and peaches. Blend the mixture until it is creamy and smooth. You can strain the mixture if you want to remove the small seeds or you can drink it as it is.

2. Banana Ginger Smoothie

This banana and ginger smoothie can sooth digestive problems and can prevent nausea and heartburn.

1 banana, sliced

1 tbsp honey

¾ cup vanilla yogurt

½ tsp freshly grated ginger

Makes 2 servings

Blend the yogurt first then add the ginger and banana. Continue to blend until it is smooth. Sweeten the drink with honey. Add ice last if you want a cool drink. Serve.

3. Blueberry, banana and green tea smoothie

It is full of antioxidants and has natural caffeine which can give you an energy boost.

2 tbsp water

2 tsp honey

Half banana

1 green tea bag

1 ½ cups frozen blueberries

¾ cup vanilla soy milk

Makes 1 servings

Boil water and soak the tea bag in a bowl for 3 minutes. Add the honey and stir to combine. Place the berries, milk and bananas in the blender and process until it is smooth. Slowly pour the tea to the blender then process until smooth. Add the ice then pulse few more times before serving.

4. Fruit breakfast smoothie

This breakfast smoothie is loaded with nutrient rich fruits.

1 cup frozen raspberries

¼ cup frozen pitted cherries

1 ½ tbsp honey

1 tsp ground flaxseed

¾ cup chilled almond ilk

2 tsp grated ginger

2 tsp lemon juice

Makes 2 servings

Pour the almond milk into the blender. Blend the ginger and flaxseed first before adding the fruits. Blend until smooth. Add the lemon juice to add taste. Add the ice last then blend again. Pour into 2 glasses and serve.

5. Tropical papaya perfection

This smoothie is as thick as a milk shake and has a strong tropical taste.

1 papaya, cut into chunks

½ cup fresh pineapple chunks

1 tsp coconut extract

1 cup fat free yogurt

½ cup ice

1 tsp ground flaxseed

Makes 1 serving

Place the fruits in a blender and process for a minute. Add the coconut extract and yogurt. Pulse few times then add the ice. Blend for few seconds until it is smooth then serve.

6. Apricot Mango Smoothie

The lemon adds a tangy flavor to the sweet smoothie. This is a perfect drink during a hot weather.

6 apricots, peeled and chopped

1 cup milk

¼ tsp vanilla extract

2 ripe mangos

4 tsp fresh lemon juice

8 ice cubes

Makes 2 servings

Place the mangoes, milk, vanilla extract, lemon juice and apricots in the blender. Blend for 8 seconds. Add the ice then process for 5 seconds. Pour in a glass then garnish with lemon zest if desired.

7. Spinach smoothie with avocado and apple

The avocado in this green smoothie makes it creamy without adding any dairy.

1 ½ cups apple juice

1 apple, chopped and cored

2 cups chopped spinach

Half avocado

Makes 2 servings

Combine the apple juice, spinach, apple and avocado in the blender. Puree until you have a smooth consistency. Add more water until you reach the desired consistency.

8. Collard green smoothie with lime and mango

This healthy smoothie taste sweet and tangy thanks to the fruits.

2 tbsp fresh lime juice

1 ½ cups frozen mango

2 cups stemmed and chopped collard greens

1 cup green grapes

Makes 2 servings

Mix the water and collard greens in a blender. Add the mango and grapes then puree until it is smooth. Blend for a minute then add the water until you have the desired consistency.

9. Watermelon smoothie wonder

Watermelon is a summer delight favorite. Remember to purchase seedless watermelon or remove the seeds before blending to ensure that you have a smooth consistency.

2 cups chopped watermelon

2 cups ice

¼ cup fat free milk

Makes 2 servings

Mix the milk and watermelon. Blend the mixture for several seconds. Add the ice and blend for a longer time. Add ice then pulse for few seconds. Serve in a glass.

10. Berry good workout smoothie

This is a great pre-workout smoothie that can give you energy for your workouts.

1 ½ cup chopped strawberries

½ cup raspberries

1 tsp fresh lemon juice

1 cup blueberries

2 tbsp honey

½ cup ice cubes

Makes 1 serving

Add all of the ingredients in the blender except for the ice. Blend until smooth. Add the ice then pulse for 6 seconds before pouring in a glass.

11. Tropical green smoothie

This tropical flavored smoothie contains the right amount of fruits and vegetables. It is also rich in nutrients and antioxidants.

2 cups fresh spinach

1 cup mango

2 bananas

2 cups water

1 cup pineapple

Makes 2 servings

Place the 2 cups of greens in the blender then process. Add the water and blend again until there are no chunks left. Add the fruits then blend again until it is smooth. Pour in a glass then serve.

12. Spinach, coconut and grape smoothie

The spinach, coconut and grapes give off an exotic and tropical taste. You can drink this smoothie as a recovery drink.

1 cup seedless green grapes

½ cup ice

1 cup baby spinach

¼ cup coconut milk

Makes 1 serving

Blend all of the ingredients in the blender until it is smooth. You can add the ice at the end of the process and blend it again few times before pouring in a glass.

13. Kale smoothie with pineapple and banana

Kale is very nutritious. Pineapple and banana add natural sweetness to the smoothie.

½ cup coconut milk

1 ½ cups pineapple, chopped

2 cups chopped kale

1 ripe banana, chopped

Makes 2 servings

Combine all of the ingredients in the blender and process until smooth. Add ice if desired.

14. Soy smoothie

This soy smoothie is rich in protein and probiotics which can effectively curb your cravings.

1 cup soy milk

½ cup corn flakes cereal

½ cup frozen blueberries

1 frozen bananas, sliced

Makes 1 serving

Mix the ingredients in the blender and process for 20 seconds. Add water or ice if desired then blend it for another 15 seconds.

15. Mango madness

Mangoes are rich in disease fighting compounds that can improve your immune system. Its natural sweet flavor can also satisfy your sweet tooth.

1 cup pineapple chunks

1 large mango, peeled and chopped

Crushed ice

1 cup yogurt

1 ripe banana, sliced

Makes 2 servings

Combine everything except for the ice. Blend until it is smooth. Add the iced at the end of the process then for few seconds.

Conclusion

Thank you again for purchasing this book!

I hope this book was able to help you to understand the smoothie diet.

The next step is to make delicious smoothies.

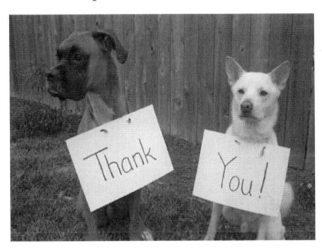

Finally, if you enjoyed this book, then I'd like to ask you for a favor, would you be kind enough to leave a review for this book on Amazon? It'd be greatly appreciated!

Thank you and good luck!

Printed in Great Britain
by Amazon